DREAMING BEYOND YOUR DIAGNOSIS

A 10 step manual on living a successful life with a disability

JAS WALKIN

DEDICATION

To My Mother:

Linda Lynette Higgs-Walkin

"Mama"

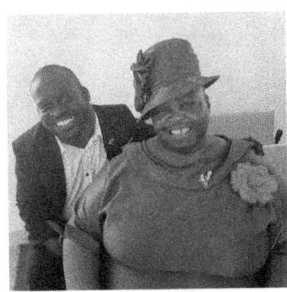 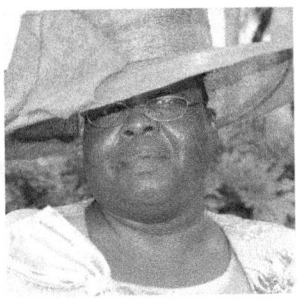

If you were to ask most people "who is the greatest influence on your life?", they would say their mom. My answer is no different; however, I must add that my Mama's role in my life was amplified because, without a manual, she had to figure out how to raise a child with special needs in an era where information, resources, and understanding were scarce. Mama demonstrated to me that a good mother is the last person to abandon her child, regardless of the challenges. As I wrote the reflections and examples in this book, it was as if I was reliving the experiences which have profoundly shaped my life and character. When I began to document our memories, I was overwhelmed with emotions of gratitude and a renewed appreciation for the woman God gave to me as a mother. Even though I lost her in January 2019, her impact on my life and my ability to not just dream but to live mydreams without excuses or 'settle for mediocrity' as she would say can never be lost. To this end, I chose to further honour her legacy through the publication of this book in the hope that it would encourage another mother to inspire hope and motivate her child's desire to Dream Beyond their Diagnosis.

CONTENTS

Dedication .... *iii*

Introduction 1

Step 1: Like it or Not the Child is Yours 5

Step 2: Parents: You Must Become Your
Child's Number One Advocate 11

Step 3: Know the Difference Between
Nurturing & Creating Codependency 19

Step 4: Know When to Cut the Navel Cord 23

Step 5: Surround Yourself with People
Who See the Gift in Your Child 29

Step 6: You are different. Accept It! 35

Step 7: Dealing with Adversities 41

Step 8: Creating Your Own Space 51

Step 9: Face your Fears with Faith 59

Step 10: Discovering the Best Kept
Secrets of Getting Ahead 69

INTRODUCTION

Regardless of our distinctive individuality, we were all created by one sovereign God who has designed us for a specific purpose. This might be difficult for some people to believe, especially those born with a disability or diagnosed with a special need which might put them at a disadvantage to living life to the fullest compared to persons without disability. From my personal experience: I was born with Cerebral Palsy (though never officially diagnosed), I can tell you that it is not easy growing up with a disability. It is more difficult when you have to do it in a community that has not been greatly exposed to persons with physical or cognitive disabilities, or who still have the primitive belief that the circumstance of your birth was the result of some curse or wrongdoing your family did in the past.

Although advocacy and education about persons with disabilities have been amplified in the twenty-first century, it has not eliminated the discrimination, resistance to inclusion, and slow implementation of laws creating equal opportunities for persons with special needs to live successful lives. Most importantly, the everyday challenges these individuals and their families have to go through to survive, much less dream about living a successful meaningful life have not been eliminated.

I wrote this book as a manual for these special people and their support systems to provide them with practical steps and examples from my life and experiences have allowed me to not just dream but live those dreams. Yes, you have a disability or a diagnosis but that doesn't have to be a death sentence. You will have challenges and be oppressed at times but you have to keep dreaming. You might be bullied but you must endure and believe that you will overcome.

In reality, all special needs diagnoses are not the same. Even my diagnosis of Cerebral Palsy has varied symptoms. I have spinal curvature (neck area), a history of epileptic seizures, and brain injury creating involuntary movements but thankfully no cognitive impairments or learning disability. The point I am trying to make is that we do not have uniform experiences. Therefore, not every experience or piece of advice shared in this book will speak directly to every diagnosis or special needs situation but the lessons can be applied. I can promise you that every parent with a special needs child as well as anyone who has been counted out or felt as if their present condition has placed them at a disadvantage in life will find encouragement within the pages of this book. My life has not been a bed of roses but I learned to dream and work to live those dreams, and if I can do it, so can you!

Disclaimer: While the majority of this book is geared towards those with a diagnosis or impairment, you will find that the first four steps or chapters are geared toward parents and caregivers who play a vital role in raising every child and more so in those with disabilities or special needs.

STEP 1:

LIKE IT OR NOT THE CHILD IS YOURS

When two people come together, and a child is concieved, whether it was planned or just an accident (like some people believe). Once that child comes to term and is delivered, he or she is yours and becomes your responsibility. Just as children don't get to choose their parents, parents are not given the luxury of choosing the child(ren) God gives them. For the record, I am not referring to the mothers who make certain poor choices during pregnancy which have the potential to alter the physical and mental characteristics of their foetus although I believe God has the final say in that regard. Nevertheless, the child God gave you is the one He purposed that you should have.

That being said, it is a challenge raising children who don't have a disability so it is easy to understand it is more difficult to raise a child living with a disability. The moment you realize something is wrong with your child, can be a very terrifying one. To hear doctors or specialists say that your child has been diagnosed with Downs Syndrome, Autism, Cerebral Palsy, an Intellectual Disability, ADHD, Traumatic Brain Injury, Medical Disabilities, or Mobility Disabilities is not an easy pill to swallow. Immediately, you would think about all the dreams and desires you had for this child and how this new reality or diagnosis will impact their life. You might begin to feel helpless, especially if the support and therapeutic services necessary for their development are not readily available. Nevertheless, the child is yours.

Cheer Up!

Additionally, you might develop feelings of guilt foolishly questioning every decision you took in the past or during pregnancy; nevertheless, the child is yours. You are feeling so frustrated with the situation and may be doing it all alone, especially the mother who doesn't have the support of family and close circle of friends as a support system. Listen to me: cheer up! This child that is presenting several challenges to you at the moment, could also become your greatest gift and life lesson. God chose you for this gift even if it came in a wrinkled gift wrap. As much as children are to be taught by parents, they also teach parents valuable lessons as well.

It is your responsibility to love that child beyond measure and reassure them every day that they matter to you. My mother Linda (whom I called Mama) was a great example of unconditional love irrespective of the diagnosis. I could only imagine her concerns when she saw that I was not developing at a pace equal to that of my peers. Nevertheless, besides the stories she shared with me, my very first memories of my Mama was her love, devotion, and assistance she gave me as a child. When I looked into her eyes, I saw love and joy. Every time she assisted me with a task that I should have been able to do but couldn't because of my disability, it was done in love not just duty.

I had several moments of low self-esteem and depression during which I questioned my place in my mother's life by asking her "Mama, are you sorry you had me? Mama, do you wish I was like other children?"

She never hesitated to reaffirm for me that I was her gift and her shining star. Additionally, she constantly reminded me of Psalm 139 in which David declared that he was fearfully and wonderfully made by his creator. Those words from the scriptures would become my reaffirmation of faith and motto every time an attack was launched on my physical appearance. In the years to follow, I can recall my mother's unwavering support and unconditional love for me, sometimes it meant protecting me from other family members who did not see me the way she did. All through my life, I have had examples of where my mother's acceptance of my condition was not used as an excuse for me not to dream but rather a motivation for her to provide me with the necessary support to be successful.

Here's the thing, as long you are in denial of your child's condition, you cannot see them as a gift and then seek to develop their gift. When you are in denial, you are limiting the possibilities for your child and delaying any available support they can receive to assist in their journey in life. Hence, making it very paramount for you as a parent, **to embrace your child for who (s)he is**. As aforementioned, whether you like it or not, the child is yours. Your child's ability to function normally or dream is based on the love and support you provide to them from the moment they take their first breath to the moment they are diagnosed and eventually their entire journey of learning to live life with a disability. When the initial shock is over, and perhaps the pity party has been concluded, you still have a child to raise. Practically, depending on the diagnosis, the experience will be different but the formula is the same. For an injured bird to fly from the nest, it must be cared for, nurtured, and most importantly, infused with confidence and a support system that convinces the bird that it is able to fly.

APPLICATION

Recite these 4 Confidence Statements daily to remind yourself that your child is a gift!

1. *(Insert your child's name)* is a blessing!
2. *Insert your child's name)* has a beautiful purpose.
3. *Insert your child's name)* matters to me and God.
4. I love *Insert your child's name)*.

REFLECTION

STEP 2:

PARENTS: YOU MUST BECOME YOUR CHILD'S NUMBER ONE ADVOCATE

Once you have accepted that your child has a disability or special need, the next step is to act. In my capacity working in Special Needs Education in a small developing Caribbean country, I am all too familiar with the realities facing parents of children diagnosed with special needs. For some parents, after the diagnosis, it is even more depressing because they have an understanding of what the disability is but there is no support system to assist them with helping their children live a normal life. Even in countries where there are services and facilities providing support to special needs children, there is always a need for more advocacy, especially in regards to greater access to inclusive education, physical and therapeutic services, occupational, speech, and language therapists.

There is a constant fight and advocacy for the rights of children with special needs to be afforded the same access to the opportunities afforded to their counterparts. However, there is no greater advocate for a child with a disability than the parent. Simply put, **you are your child's greatest defender and advocate**. Besides protecting them from being taken advantage of, you must develop an advocacy type spirit from his/her early days that makes your child know that you are their number one cheerleader.

A TEACHER'S NIGHTMARE

For example, I am grateful that my mother was a teacher. By virtue of her profession alone, she was trained to be an advocate for children in general. Nevertheless, when she herself was faced with the realities of having a child with special needs, it was a different ball game. Picture this, she was a teacher on a small, underdeveloped island just benefiting from electricity four years prior to my birth. Culturally, children with physical or mental disabilities were shunned and barely acknowledged much less celebrated by their families. My mother was teaching primary school and did everything possible to teach me at home. But as expected, when I reached school age, she wanted me to receive an education like the children she had taught over the years. It was probably early in preschool when she realized the challenges I would have forming letters in a book and writing coherently.

Her fears were further heightened during Infant one when my teacher expressed frustration with not being able to assist me with basic writing skills because my disability characterized by involuntary shaking made it nearly impossible to hold a pencil to write. I remember my mother asking me several evenings after school to bring my notebook so she could see what I did in school but was disappointed when she realized my book did not have much in it. However, she could ask me any lesson or question related to what I was being taught and I was able to recite it back to her. Mama was discouraged and further discouraged when some of her own colleagues and neighbours felt that she wanted too much for me or was pushing me too much. At age four I remember adults telling my mother "Linda, you have to accept that Jas is not like other children and you need to accept he has a disability". The problem was not my mother's denial of my limitations; the problem was she was not prepared to allow my physical limitations to impede my ability to learn.

What did mama do? My mama kept fighting and kept insisting that I receive a general education because in her words "there was shaking in my shoulder, but not in my head". She built a support system that convinced me that I belonged in a general education classroom (especially considering there were no special needs education classrooms at the school) and constantly pushed me to tough it out. She became a backbone for me on days when I wanted to quit, on days when I was bullied, on days when my teachers did not understand what I was feeling; Mama was there. I witnessed her standing up for me to her colleagues as well as the Principal when the need arose.

Even when I entered high school, there were a few examples when my mama had to turn into 'Mama Bear'. For instance, Technical Drawing was timetabled for male students in my school from seventh to ninth grade. One day my teacher gave the class an assignment which my motor skills and physical limitations prevented me from doing. When I tried to explain to the teacher that I was having difficulty completing the drafting assignment, he got angry and physically punished me (corporal punishment was legal at that time in schools). I walked out of his class and walked up the hill to my mother's school (the primary and secondary schools were adjacent to each other) and explained my frustration about being chastised and punished for something that I physically could not do. She asked me to stop crying and to go back to school. My mother scheduled a meeting with the teacher explaining my history and struggles just to make it to secondary school and why he was wrong for what transpired. I never experienced another incident like that in my high school tenure.

It takes a village

Under normal circumstances, raising a child should be a village exercise comprising support from family, public services, and community in general. With raising a special needs child you need the support of the community and your advocacy. There will be times when you feel alone and as if no one is in your corner. There will be times when the system denies you and your child the services and assistance necessary for them to function like children without disabilities. This is not because they are against supporting your situation but rather because they are not prepared to help develop the special gift you have been given. What do you do? Continue to advocate; continue to find ways of arming yourself and those who form your support circle with information as you continue to build a conducive environment for the growth and successful development of your child.

Most importantly, in the face of adversity, demonstrate to your child that although life will not be a bed of roses, you won't settle to "make the best of it". Through your advocacy, fight, and constantly push for a better living, an enjoyable and fulfilling life for your child. Teach them that indeed, they belong to this universe, and there is a gift in them to be developed and explored, a gift that may one day positively impact the lives of other people. This is what my mother did for me. She not only provided me with unconditional love and support but through her advocacy, she developed in me an attitude of achievement and helped to develop a fighting spirit within me. A fighting spirit that helped me defeat bullies, push doors open, and demand seats at tables once considered too high for a man like me.

I share these experiences with you because my mother was my superhero without superpowers. I am confident that if you want your child to have stories similar to mine, you will find ways of becoming their superhero. I believe as you read this book, you already have what it takes to be your child's hero; you just need to activate these things. If you don't remember anything I wrote in this chapter, please remember this; **you cannot ask other people to believe in the future and the possibilities of your child more than you do**. You must be the captain of their dream and steer them until they can steer themselves; remember the famous quote "the captain is the last to leave the ship".

APPLICATION

Recite these 4 Confidence Statements in the mirror daily.

1. I am my child's best advocate.
2. I am blessed and I am bold.
3. I will speak up, even if my voice shakes.
4. I will confront issues with love and grace.

REFLECTION

STEP 3:

KNOW THE DIFFERENCE BETWEEN NURTURING & CREATING CODEPENDENCY

You will hear me repeat throughout this book the statement: **every special need or disability presents a unique set of challenges**. However, the advice and examples given in each step in this book are relatable to the parents and their children who actually have had to live the experiences of raising a child with a disability. That being said, this step is a bit complex and varies significantly based on the nature of the disability. One of the most important but overlooked steps in accepting your child's disability and responding to it, is the recognition of your child's 'ability' in their 'disability'.

Parents often make the mistake of only focusing on what their special needs child cannot do and ways to make accommodations for those disabilities and the circumstances they create. Instead, the approach equally needs to be focused on the abilities they have. More importantly, learn to develop those abilities while still nurturing them and supporting them in the areas of their life that their disability has created a necessity for assistance.

For example, I was born with Cerebral Palsy, displaying symptoms of underdeveloped motor skills, spinal curvature (my neck), problems with coordination, epileptic seizures, and involuntary movements, but no learning disability or cognitive impairments. Immediately, my mother recognized that despite my physical developmental delays, I possessed a very high functioning brain. Hence, she prepared herself to support me in my physical activities or those tasks requiring the discipline of my motor skills. She assisted with buttoning my shirt and buckling my pants until I was able to do them myself. She opened packages for me, tied my shoelaces, and understood it was not pampering or spoiling me. On the other hand, she made no excuses for me in regards to my cognitive skills or sharp and quick oratory skills. Additionally, she taught me to read even though early on I could not write.

Nurturing versus dependency

My mother understood that she needed to nurture me to not become dependent on her forever. Instead, she fostered her support in a climate in which I knew that I needed to be as independent as I could and only ask for help when extremely necessary. I know it is easy for you to say "Jas, you don't understand my situation or the challenges my child is facing" and maybe you are right. However, think about these questions; have you ever asked yourself what abilities your child has? What have I taught my child to do for himself or herself? When was the last time I observed a new growth and development in my child? These questions are important because you have to find a balance between providing the necessary support and nurturing your child needs and raising them to be as independent as possible. As I said before, this approach will vary based on the nature of your child's disability, as we are cognizant that their physical abilities and development depends on their intellectual abilities.

Nevertheless, wherever there is an opportunity to teach your child to be self-reliant, you must do so. Nurture and support them with the belief that they will grow up to lead successful, independent lives away from you one day. Hence, where possible, equip them with the skills and attitude that there might come a day when 'mama will not be there to catch me when I fall'. It may be scary but you can do it.

APPLICATION

List 4 things you can do right now to prepare your child for a life of full or partial independence.

_____

_____

_____

_____

STEP 4:

KNOW WHEN TO CUT THE NAVEL CORD

In truth, this step is almost a postscript to step three *(3) Know the Difference Between Nurturing & Creating* Co-dependency. Additionally, I even considered including it within step three (3) but I felt it might be lost. So, here it goes.

You have done a great job figuring out how to support your child and still discover their abilities. You have built confidence in them as well as reassure them that you see them as a gift just waiting to be fully unwrapped. What is next? Caribbean people have an expression; "you have to cut the navel cord". Its translation is as follows: there comes a time after you have raised your children and provided them with all the support and guidance you can, you have to let them go and spread their wings and live their lives. This is difficult for most parents especially mothers who spent much time caring for their child. So it is not hard to imagine how much more difficult it is for a parent of a special needs child to **release them into the world**.

Cut the Cord

Firstly, this ability to 'cut the cord' does not happen overnight. You must first take small steps, like allowing them to fail at doing certain tasks until they are strong enough to do it themselves. Or when you discover they can learn and retain what they learn, take steps to include them in a learning environment among their peers either in inclusive education or special education classroom depending on the resources and services available. For example, after my mother realized that I had a normal functioning brain, she began preparing me for school. She was scared out of her wits to let me be schooled with my peers, especially being cognizant of the cultural stance and perception of special needs children at that time. She walked me to preschool every day until she felt comfortable allowing her past students and other family members to do it. She visited my class as often as possible and questioned me about how I was treated by my teacher. This continued until she realized I was going to be ok without her presence for periods of the day.

Secondly, my mother's bravery was further illustrated when it was time for me to leave primary school (the same school she taught at) and enter secondary school. Imagine her fears as she was preparing me for secondary school; this child that has been with her through pre-school and primary school, the child who has had lunch with her five days a week for eight years will be moving onto another level of education. Then, came her biggest challenge; watching me prepare to travel to another country for college. The morning my mother left me in Nassau, Bahamas to return to the Turks & Caicos Islands, I felt the cord being cut. When she got home, she called and told me how difficult it was for her to leave me that day, and subsequently, she was sick for weeks requiring a DNC. One of her friends told her that her symptoms were similar to what a woman goes through after birth. That was because she was letting me go for a big step in my life's journey.

Thirdly, you have to trust other people with the care of your child at times. Why? Because as great as you are, you are not an island to yourself. The summer after my first year in primary school, mama and I were frustrated with the challenges I encountered during my first year in an inclusive education classroom. We visited one of her friends, Maureen (also a teacher and a name you will read about several times in this book), on another island in the archipelago and while at her home, I saw my mother's trust in other people put to the test. After sharing our experiences with Maureen, she allowed her to take me into her classroom at home and teach me how to write. I was a coward and began to cry for mama. At that moment, I did not need mama, instead, I needed tough love from a stranger. Despite my outbursts, moaning, and cries for mama, my mother had to stay away and trust Maureen to teach me some valuable lessons (details to be shared later) that would forever change my life.

Moreover, it is unrealistic for you to believe that you will be with your child twenty-four seven (24/7) or that you are the only support or guidance they will need in life. If you reflect on my previous examples in this chapter, you will recall the process my mother went through before getting to a point where she could trust other people with me. At first, it was letting family members babysit me, then trusting my teachers to educate me, my classmates to accept and embrace me, and then trusting me to know when I was strong enough to leave her nest and spread my wings.

APPLICATION

List 4 milestones in your child's development that may give you confidence to increase their independence.

1. _____

2. _____

3. _____

4. _____

REFLECTION

STEP 5:

SURROUND YOURSELF WITH PEOPLE WHO SEE THE GIFT IN YOUR CHILD

I believe you can tell by now that the book has been written as a step by step manual to gradually prepare the parent to develop a special needs child to believe in themselves and it is proceeding to focus on the child giving advice supported by personal experiences. That being said, after becoming an advocate for your child, nurtured them into a strong confident individual, you still need the support of others. The support I speak of is not just for your child but also for you. Rearing a child with a disability is not easy even when done by a united couple. You will need the support of family and friends. You will also need mental and physical breaks from parenting which could be in the form of social events with other adults, vacations, or conversations about topics other than experiences raising a special needs child.

Surround Yourself with People Who See the Gift in Your Child

When you choose to be around or look to people for outside help or support, make sure those individuals see your child as the gift you have grown to see him/her as. Make sure those people value your dedication to developing a successful child and will contribute to the mental, spiritual, and physical capacity needed to raise your special needs child. When I look back at my life and the many individuals who touched my life, I must say I was blessed. My mother always surrounded herself and by extension me with positive people who encouraged her to develop my abilities. One of the first persons I can recall positively impacting my life from my mother's circle of friends was my Godmother Patricia Hamilton. My Goddie Pat spoiled me and made me the apple of her eye. She took special care of me and provided me a safe haven outside of my mother's nest for many years. The same can be said for my surrogate mother Yvette Gardiner (I call her Nana) who from my birth decided to love me unconditionally and always made me feel as special and sometimes even more special than her own children.

Another individual who positively changed my life was Maureen. This was the woman who first introduced me to tough love. In the summer of 1989, Maureen helped me to come face to face with one of my greatest enemies, self-pity (I will elaborate in a later step) and challenged me to think beyond my physical limitations. If that was not enough, Maureen also gave me the proper tools to be able to physically put letters on paper, and she taught me that my disability was not an excuse to be an academic failure especially when I was gifted with a brain that could learn. There was Linda Williams, Lillian Been Boyce, Beatrice Skippings, Jane Williams, Henrietta Delancy, and Punchetta Taylor and so many others who in one way or the other found means of motivating me or were there for me during critical moments of my life. There is a list as long as the river Nile of people who my mother brought into my life throughout the years who in their own way helped to develop me and helped me to identify the gift and purpose God had designed for me to fulfil.

What am I trying to say? **You don't have to teach your child how to dream alone.** Find the right type of help from people and create an environment and culture for your child to be raised in. Not only will this increase the possibilities for the positive growth and development of your child, but it will also create a sense of appreciation for people and the desire to serve others. Perhaps it is why when the opportunity came for me to choose a career path, I chose a path of public service. My decision to be a public servant was as a result of the call I felt on my life to give back to people the way so many people had given to me.

APPLICATION

List 4 people (other than you) that you would like to establish stronger relationships with in order to create a stronger village for your child.

1. _____

2. _____

3. _____

4. _____

THIS SECTION OF THE BOOK SPEAKS SPECIFICALLY TO THE SPECIAL NEEDS CHILD OR INDIVIDUAL.

As previously established, my purpose in writing this book was to provide a step-by-step manual for parents of children with a disability as well as for the individual with the disability. The remaining steps therefore, are geared especially towards the individual with the disability or special need.

REFLECTION

STEP 6:

YOU ARE DIFFERENT. ACCEPT IT!

One of the fundamental reasons why I believe in the creation story and the existence of an all-knowing, all-powerful God is because human beings and the individuality each one possesses could only be orchestrated by a supreme God. God demonstrates His awesomeness every time a child is born with distinct characteristics. That being said, the reasons so many people want to be like others is beyond my comprehension. Nevertheless, I was one of those individuals who once desired to be someone else and who did not understand why I was created differently. No, I am not referring to my unique DNA; instead, I am referring to me being born with Cerebral Palsy (though not officially diagnosed as a child) and the physical challenges that accompany it.

For you to better understand my struggle with accepting myself, let me share this reflection with you. I was about four years old when I began to realize that my childhood would be difficult. Why? Because when I looked in the mirror, I saw at that time an imperfect human being. I saw a little boy that looked handicapped with an uncontrollable shaking problem, a neck that leaned on the side (due to Spinal Curvature), and that was displeased with his physical appearance. I would always look at the boys my age or childhood friends and wish that I looked like them. To me, they were *normal*; they stood upright, they could use both of their hands and moved confidently. No one questioned their physical ability or endurance, and certainly, no one had a reason to make fun of their appearance. When they walked into a room, no one jeered at them or stared at their physical indifference. These feelings developed low self-esteem in me. I would always ask my mama "why did God have to make me this way?" I would bombard her with "why can't I be like other children?" Even though my mother did an awesome job reassuring me that God knew what He was doing when He made me different, it was no comfort to me.

As I grew older, I became more and more conscious about my physical appearance. Determined to be like others, I would pray every night for God to make me like everybody else. I could not understand that God had done me a favour. I could not understand that God had created me this way to set me apart from all the other children my age because I was a gift only to be discovered and developed. Moreover, I could not understand that sometimes for you to be different, God has to make you different.

Reality

My self-esteem and self-acceptance began to change because of three realizations. The first realization was this; any time you feel you have an unfair situation in life, there are others with worse conditions. In the early 1990s, I attended a Special Needs Symposium in Providenciales (sister island in the Turks & Caicos Archipelago). Most importantly, on that trip, I got a reality check. Up to that point in my life, I had always viewed myself as a person who was physically disabled. However, when I attended the sessions at that conference and I met people with Down's syndrome, one leg, no legs, no arms, blind, deaf, mute, and several behavioural disorders, I began to really question myself and consider whether or not I really had a disability. I went back to my room after the first night and offered an apology prayer to God. Here I was believing that injustice in this life was done to me because I have a shaking problem and could not effectively use my right hand.

I said, "God I am sorry for being so ungrateful". I am complaining about the inability to use my right hand but I saw people with no right hand. I do not like my head being leaned on the side but some people could not have a normal conversation with me. Some people had eyes but could not see, ears but could not hear. I began to appreciate God for His creation and the wonderful work He had done in my life. My mind began to meditate on a scripture my mother had instilled in me from birth, "I will praise thee for I was fearfully and wonderfully made, Marvellous are thy works Oh God." Psalm 139:14 I began to tell myself "**You are different. Accept it and embrace it**". Gradually, how I looked began to matter less and less. God made me and called me perfect, so who am I to complain about His marvellous works?

This brings me to my second realization; once you have accepted that you are different, **it matters less if people accept you or not**. Too often we project our low self-esteem onto others asking them to do something for us we have not done for ourselves. The moment I began embracing who I was, I decreased the number of pity parties I threw for myself and stopped expecting people around me to feel sorry for me.

Finally, after you embrace that you are different, **be prepared to live, and be treated differently**. Your experiences in your life will significantly be shaped by your disability or special need. The truth of the matter is this; the world often is not accommodating to those of us who were created differently or physically challenged, thus making it difficult for us to complete certain tasks. My experience has taught me that institutions and leaders make far too many decisions only concentrating on how to empower the strong and not enough time seeking ways of protecting and empowering the vulnerable members of society. Hence, prepare to be an advocate for yourself and accept the need to develop a fighting spirit. People who are different are treated differently so we also learn to think and live differently. Why? Because failure to do this will severely hinder your ability to successfully deal with adversity.

APPLICATION

Recite these 4 Confidence Statements in the mirror daily.

1. My life matters!
2. I have a great purpose!
3. I am unstoppable!
4. Nothing or anyone will hold me back!

STEP 7:

DEALING WITH ADVERSITIES

First and foremost, once you enter this world and make it through infancy and childhood into adulthood, you will face adversities in life. There is no escaping it because each day we live presents new challenges that we must deal with. That being said, if an individual born with no physical or cognitive delays or impairments is expected to face and deal with their adversities in their lifetime, for the individual born with a disability, it will be double the adversities because you will have the regular challenges life throws at everyone, and then you will have those challenges you encounter because of your disability and the circumstances it has created for you. Double the adversities means you need to double efforts to face and defeat them. In this chapter, through the experiences shared, I intend to offer some advice on how a special needs individual can respond to adversities and come out victorious.

If you missed it in the previous steps or chose to jump straight to this chapter (that is allowed), my special need was characterized by the symptoms of Cerebral Palsy; Spinal Curvature, seizures, involuntary physical movements, weak muscles, and underdeveloped motor skills and stiff finger joints. With those characteristics in mind, let me first take you to my first problem; starting primary school. I was terrified to go to school because I felt like I did not belong. This terror would be compounded by frustration when my teacher, despite her best efforts, could not assist me with writing basic alphabet letters in my notebook. I so badly wanted to do this especially when I saw the excitement and doggy stickers my classmates received when they completed their writing assignments. I can recall the frustration even at age four trying to hold my yellow pencil and wanting badly to control my shaking so my pencil point would not break. It always broke, and with every broken pencil, my frustration grew.

Not to mention the pressure, nervousness and discomfort I experienced watching these stronger kids watch me as if something was wrong with me (and something did feel wrong) while my teacher used every skill she possessed trying to reach me. At the end of infant one (as the school system called it), school had no purpose for me and I had no desire to return. I told my mama exactly how I felt and fought passionately with her to sympathize with me and agree with my perspective; I was not cut out for integrated education or school in general.

The only thing I had on my young, inexperienced mind was quitting. Although mama was frustrated herself, she knew that she could not let me quit, and give up on the possibility of receiving a comprehensive elementary education. Hence, with our backs against the wall, I discovered one of the first ways of dealing with adversity; **you have to acknowledge it and vent to someone who understands** your experiences and can possibly help you overcome them.

This brings me to the summer of 1989, and a woman named Maureen Williams. I believe God placed her in my life at the most critical junction. Maureen was stern and straight forward and I was terrified of her, not understanding how this woman who appeared to me to be so mean and cold was still able and determined to extend so much affection towards me. Hence, you can imagine my perplexity when mama took me to Grand Turk (the capital island in the Turks & Caicos Islands) to Maureen's house in the summer of 1989. After eavesdropping on their conversation and concluding that Maureen was now fully brought up to speed with my frustration during my first academic school year, I began anticipating that my summer was about to take a different turn.

When Maureen took me to her laundry room where she had a classroom set up, I mentally prepared for a repeat performance of my infant one teacher with an attitude of "here we go again" and "why don't these people accept that I cannot write?". Fortunately for me, I was in for a rude awakening. Maureen not only proceeded to teach me how to write, but she also taught me several valuable lessons about dealing with adversities as a child with a physical limitation.

Lesson # 1: You Can't Change How You Were Created

When Maureen saw that I was intimidated by her presence and her attempt to guide my hands to form the letters on my notebook; - I was nervous and crying. She paused and asked me to calm down. She began to question me about why I was so nervous and shaking more than my natural involuntary movements constituted. I told her that my nervousness and fear was based on my desire for people to not look at me and see me as different. Maureen took me by the hands, sat me down and spoke these words to me: "Jas, you look different because God designed you differently. Can you change how you were born? Can you change your physical condition and appearance? Will crying change how you look?" She and I answered the questions simultaneously and consecutively: no, no, and no. Subsequently, Maureen continued to bolster my self-confidence and acceptance of who I was and what I was created to be during that summer. This experience allowed me to not only become aware of my self-worth but also to begin to celebrate my indifference and dream about things every other child would dream about. However, with a clear understanding that how I achieve those dreams would **require some adjustments and a commitment to always be willing to put in overtime**.

Lesson # 2: The Sympathy Line is Long & You are Not in Front

Another lesson Maureen taught me about dealing with adversity is that the world owes you nothing and there are other people ahead of you waiting for sympathy. What will you do? Join the line or fight for your place in the hardworking line? I can recall the exact words Maureen said to me, explaining the coldness of the world and how I needed to toughen up if I truly intend to make my mark. Her words to me were: "Jas, if you are looking for sympathy from people because of how you look, you had better think again. The sympathy line is long and you are not in the front". At that moment, I felt the last bit of self-pity and entitlement leave my spirit and mental frame. If you are going to have any chance of overcoming your adversities as a special needs individual, you must be prepared to live in a cold, selfish world where strong people often compensate for their weaknesses by trying to take advantage of weaker and vulnerable people. Knowing this, you must **develop a strong backbone and determined spirit** which is not easily broken. Believe me, this spirit will take you through life.

Lesson # 3: Bullies will be a part of your life, but don't let them take control

After Maureen explained to me that I had no choice in my biological design and that I needed not to look for sympathy for the way I looked physically during 1989summer holiday. A few years had passed and I was growing in confidence but was now dealing with another adversity. I asked her how I should handle one of the biggest challenges any child can face; bullying by both adults and children who found joy in intimidating me and constantly reaffirming my insecurities about being physically challenged and that I did not belong to this universe, much less entitled to a dream. Maureen asked me to describe for her what the nature of my bullying was and after I explained to her how I felt when I was called derogatory names and slurs which often escalated to physical harm being threatened and extended towards me, she said three things to me that once more changed my life and approach to people who tried bullying me. Maureen said, "(1) Jas, your name is not what you are called, rather what you answer to, (2) people think of others what they are themselves, and (3) it takes two fools to make a quarrel when one can always end it". It should be noted that number three was the last principle I mastered in life.

At the end of this conversation, I was equipped with mental weapons to defend myself. I developed a very sharp tongue filled with fire and brimstone ready to defend myself when I was teased. Although my victories did not come overnight, as the years went by in primary school, I learned how to cope with bullying and found out that I was frustrating them because though they were physically stronger than me, I was mentally stronger than them. Furthermore, if you think dealing with bullies in primary school was difficult, high school bullies took it to another level. My first year in high school were some of my worst days dealing with bullies because the strategies I used as a coping mechanism in primary school quickly proved to be ineffective. I was dealing with bullies who physically accosted me and often tried to take away my lunch money. Their constant verbal attacks during my grade seven year began to erode eight years of progress of confidence-building by my mother and people like Maureen had assisted me in developing.

I began to revert to my shell of insecurity and wanted to quit. I even skipped school for a few days behind my mother's back in my attempt to avoid the adversity of high school bullying. When my mother discovered my truancy and the West Indian whopping that followed, she sat and explained to me that quitting was not an option. She then jumped into superhero mode, and reminded me of what was at stake and forced me to reflect on my journey thus far, and how we overcome the adversities of the past together . Hence, believing things would get better and drawing from my past well of resilience, I survived my first year of high school. However, I had four more years to go and I needed a new strategy to not just complete secondary school, but also find a way to actually enjoy my high school experience.

Thankfully, at the start of grade eight, I went through a personality transformation that inadvertently gave me the formula to defeat my bullies in high school once and for all. I began my second year in secondary school with a new attitude; the attitude was "I am here to stay and God help the man who will stand in the way of my education". This attitude also ignited a newfound self-confidence and the belief that I am handsome and I'm God's gift to the girls in high schools. Additionally, I began to idolize WWF wrestling superstar "The Heartbreak Kid" (HBK) Sexy Boy Shawn Michaels and developed an alter ego with his personality. I would walk around the school during recess with my shirt top three buttons loose and singing "I'm not your boy toy, I'm just a sexy boy". Moreover, I also became an obsessed fan of James Bond 007 movies and characterizations; hence, when I was not behaving like HBK Shawn Michaels, I was imitating confident and suave Pierce Brosnan or Sean Connery. Funny enough, my Hotmail address created from that period and still used till date is jas007hbk@hotmail.com.

When bullies saw my confidence and new swagger, their insults and intimidation began to decrease because they realized it was no longer affecting me. Instead of running away and folding up in a corner like a scared puppy, I was bold and fully embraced the new me. I had finally reached a place in my life where how I looked did not matter to me. Furthermore, I discovered powerful defence to disarm bullies who attacked my physical appearance; humour, and self-humiliation. Basically, I discovered that if I made fun of my physical appearance before bullies did or responded to their teasing with witty comebacks of the same nature, it took their ammunition away. For example, I would make statements like "my shaking makes me sexier than you and that is why you are jealous" and "is it cold in here, or is it just me?" I would even compete with bullies to see which of us would think of an insult first when we met. This approach was one of my biggest breakthroughs in life especially in overcoming the adversity of bullying. I am not saying that you have to use the same tactics I used but my point is that whatever it is, **take back control**.

Lesson # 4: Adversity Builds Character

Under normal circumstances, life is filled with adversities. Hence, as previously mentioned, as a special needs individual, you will have adversities twice that of the general population. However, how you respond to them will not only write your future but the experiences and lessons learned will build your character and resilience. This character once developed, will be instrumental to the choices you make and how you choose to see the world. Moreover, it will be a guide for how you choose to live with your disability in a world of ups and downs and twists and turns. I like to call it **Double for Your Trouble**.

APPLICATION

1) Write a name that you would give to your alter ego.
   _____

2) Write the name of 1 person that you will talk to whenever you are feeling down.

   _____

3) Think about your favorite movie character or superhero. Write 3 things that you admire about them. Apply those 3 things to yourself.

   a. _____
   b. _____
   c. _____

STEP 8:

CREATING YOUR OWN SPACE

The events that took place in the summer of 1989 changed my life in many profound ways and Maureen played a key role in many of those important moments.

Maureen spent time helping to build my self-confidence, she then turned to another task at hand; teaching me how to write despite my physical challenges. Maureen and I discovered that the regular 12b pencil was too light to sustain the pressure of my shaking and death grip every time I attempted to write; hence, the pencil point would always break. Recognizing this, she went into her husband's construction box and found the heavy-duty construction pencil and gave it to me and said "let's try this." I took the pencil and realized it had the right strength and size to sustain my shaking and started writing my first letters and words. For the rest of my primary school life and as long I needed, Maureen supplied me with large size pencils and special erasers to make it easier for me to write.

When I left Maureen's house, my life was changed in several ways and as you read earlier, I left with several lessons on dealing with adversities, and most importantly, after learning to write, I learned how to create my own space. When Maureen and I realized that the regular size pencil was ineffective, she did not insist that I make do. Instead, she found a way to make it easier for me to write, and this is what I mean when I say "Create Your Own Space." Too often people with physical challenges and disabilities struggle with being expected to perform tasks the same way their counterparts with no disabilities are expected to. Additionally, persons with disabilities frustrate themselves trying to do the impossible instead of finding new ways of doing assigned tasks.

Focus on your abilities

When you create your own space, you are finding easier ways to complete required tasks. In my scenario, my task was to write; the 12b pencil was not working so I needed a larger one. What was the goal? To write with a 12b pencil or to simply get the letters and words on the paper? This approach became my new strategy in completing difficult tasks, focusing less on my disabilities and more on my 'abilities'.

For example, early in my life, I realized that using my motor skills to hold a smooth drinking glass in my hand and turning it to my head was nearly impossible and after a few accidents, what did I do? I created my own space and used a mug or cups with handles. Hence, when I went to visit people's houses and became thirsty, I asked for the drink to be placed in a mug or cup with a handle. Additionally, my grandmother, Amedica introduced the simplicity of using straws to get the drink from the container to my mouth, again, making it easier for me to enjoy my drink.

Even when I became an adult and had to learn to live independently, I have been applying the principle of creating my own space. Consider the following practical examples:

Example #1: Because of my physical challenges and lack of coordination, I never successfully learned to tie my shoelaces. I used to love sneakers growing up but quickly realized that I could not put them on without assistance. Hence, when I started to live alone, I only bought loafers and shoes without laces. The reality is that I have to wear shoes but it is not mandatory that they have laces.

Example #2: When I entered grade nine in secondary school, I took up an interest in typewriting. Yes, the boy who once struggled to hold a pencil or pen was now at a place where he wanted to type words from a keyboard to a paper. My teacher Mrs. Davis taught us the foundations of typewriting and the numerous rules regarding the skill. She further insisted that we type with both hands on the home keys (ASDF JKL) and was prepared to disqualify persons who were not following these rules. I certainly was unable to type with all fingers on the home keys and this created a confrontation. Despite my challenges, I used the fingers (index, middle) I felt comfortable using and became one of the fastest typists in my class and certainly the most accurate one. When my teacher pointed out that I was not typing the correct way, I asked her "what is the goal of typewriting? Correctly generating words on the paper or screen or how many fingers I used to do it?"

I created my own space by typing the best and easiest way I knew how. I was so grateful for my second typewriting teacher, Valeda Gardiner, who made me so comfortable in her class and allowed me to create my own space. Additionally, she taught me to focus more on accuracy and paying attention to the manuscript I was typing rather than the style and form used to type. This experience not only allowed me to create my own space but taught me how to focus on the bigger picture in life and how to **keep being focused on goals in life and not the means to achieve them**.

Example #3: When I returned from college and began teaching, I wanted to learn how to drive. However, no one felt comfortable using their vehicle to teach me because they feared my shaking and other physical limitations would result in an accident and damage their vehicle. To be fair, their fear and concerns were justified. Nevertheless, I had an objective and I was determined to get it done. Thankfully, Yvette Handfield (one of the many women who positively contributed to my life), asked me if I was interested in learning how to drive and I told her indeed I was but explained my dilemma regarding being taught. She looked at me and said, "well I guess you need to get your own vehicle then". Not only did she tell me how to create my own space but this woman who had always shown me tough love went beyond her advice and purchased a Chevy Tracker Jeep for me and allowed me to repay in instalments.

This generous act by Yvette motivated me to learn to drive and took away excuses from those I asked to teach me. Hence, when I realized that their fear was not just their vehicle but also being in a vehicle with me at the wheel, I decided to say a prayer and began teaching myself how to drive. The vehicle was mine and I did not buy it to watch it parked in my driveway. After three days of driving on backroads in my neighbourhood, my confidence grew and I started driving. A week later, I went to the Department of Motor Vehicles to get my driver's licence on my twenty-second birthday and I have been driving ever since. I always smile when I consider that presently I own three vehicles on three different islands in the Turks & Caicos Islands Archipelago; look what the Lord has done!

Example #4: Living on my own means I have to be as independent as possible. Hence, I had to find easy ways to do things like cooking; I cook what I am able to. For example, I love corn beef because it was a staple and my father's favourite while growing up; however, I don't buy it often because I cannot open the tin it comes in. I only buy it when I have designated someone to open it for me.

In conclusion, when you accept that you have physical limitations, you must also accept the challenges that come with it. However, in accepting these challenges, you also must **accept the reality of the need to make some adjustments or living life on your terms**. From personal experience and reflection, I can tell you that there are many things I wish I could do physically, especially those tasks requiring the use of both hands, speed, accuracy, and steadiness. But at the end of the day, I live by this motto "I can only do what I can do" and continue to create my own space.

APPLICATION

1) What are 3 abilities that you have that make you proud?

   a. _____

   b. _____

   c. _____

2) Write 3 challenges that you are currently facing.

   a. _____

   b. _____

   c. _____

3) Write 3 alternative ways of solving the challenges (listed above) without the help of others.

   a. _____

   b. _____

   c. _____

REFLECTION

STEP 9:

FACE YOUR FEARS WITH FAITH

Your understanding of the next few paragraphs will be significantly based on your spiritual faith and belief in the supernatural power of God. Nevertheless, even if you do not share my Christian faith, continue to read if only to humour me until you get to a point where you can appreciate the thoughts expressed.

The best decision anyone can make in this life is to develop a relationship with God. As crazy as it might seem, my relationship with God and the foundation of my faith in Him began while I was in my mother's womb. During the last trimester of her pregnancy, she was prayed for by a woman named Amelia Been (a church sister/prayer warrior) who told her about a vision she had about my birth. She told my mom that God had revealed to her that the enemy was trying to attack her pregnancy and her life simultaneously. But she prayed for mom and anointed her stomach declaring that I was to live and be raised as Jeremiah for the rebuilding of a nation.

That story always preceded this one: the night I was born was always told to me as a reminder of why I had to be the only kid always in church. My mother said she already was stressed by my delivery exceeding the suggested due date (not abnormal) and certainly on the night I was born, her anxiety was heightened when seconds after I left her womb, it appeared as if she had lost me. Initially, I was not breathing nor responding to resuscitation. Why is the child not crying? Why is he not making any sounds? Those were the questions marinating in my mother's head at the moment I was between life and death.

A BLESSED BIRTH

Mama described for me her first vision of me; naval cord wrapped tightly around my neck, my skin colour darkened, almost blue from the oxygen deprivation, and still no sound. Mama said she began to pray and asked God to intervene, and promised Him that she would raise me in fear and reverence of Him (and believe me she did) if He spared my life. According to my mother, shortly after her prayer, she heard me crying indicating that I was alive and breathing. What this story meant for me as a child and even now as an adult was that I was nearly a stilled birth but God, in His divine will and purpose for my life, rewrote my story. This story is the foundation of my faith and relationship with God.

In the years to follow, the symptoms of Cerebral Palsy and the circumstances it created shaped my life but it also built my faith. The first experience I can recall which brought me face to face with faith was epilepsy (a symptom of Cerebral Palsy). I was four years old, getting ready for school one morning when I had an experience that rocked both me and my mother's faith and would shape my childhood for the next eight years.

My world was shaken

I can remember this specific morning as if it was yesterday. Mama was getting me ready for school and as usual, we were having our morning "sings-spiration". Mama said to me, "Jas, go and get the hairbrush". As I walked to the drawer, a funny feeling came over me. I temporarily lost consciousness while standing on my feet. Mama called my name repeatedly but I could not answer her because I was chewing my tongue and dribbling. This was the first time I experienced an epileptic seizure. When mama spun me around, I remember the fear in her eyes, as she uttered these words "Lord, what is happening to my child this morning?"

Nevertheless, I saw her faith kick in immediately when she took me in her arms and began to pray. When I reflect on the seizures I used to have, I am grateful to God that I never lost my hearing or other senses, only my speech was severely impeded. My mother held my head in her arms and began to say, "Satan, I rebuke you in the name of Jesus". She would then say to me repeatedly, "Jas, call on Jesus, say Jesus, say Jesus, etc.". Even as I write these words now, the tears are flowing down my face because I can still feel the emotions of that morning. My brain and heart wanted to say Jesus but my lips could not utter the words. But finally, once my lips had uttered the word "JESUS", the seizure was over.

As I previously mentioned, these seizures became a part of my life for the next eight years as I was placed on medication but continued to have epileptic seizures. However, I can tell you that for these eight years and countless episodes of seizures I had, at no time did the seizure continue after mother, grandmother, or any praying person said to me "say JESUS" and I uttered the name "JESUS." when . This is why I know beyond any shadow of a doubt that there is power in the name of Jesus. Jesus' name has never failed to deliver me.

Nevertheless, I struggled to develop consistent faith in God for several reasons. Firstly, I began to question why I was created with a physical disability when other children were created perfectly. Secondly, I went to every healing/prayer crusade/program that was ever formed and even placed my hands on the TV screen when tele-evangelists like Benny Hinn and Earl Roberts would pray for healing of lame and sick people but nothing happened for me.

In addition to all of this, after every episode of epilepsy, I was became depressed , sometimes feelings of suicide crept into my spirit. I would often ask my mama if I was a burden to her or if she regretted giving birth to me. As I grew older, post-seizure depression grew stronger and stronger. I asked God many times "why me?" How do you want me to trust you when you have not proven yourself to me?" So, I decided that I would not serve God until He had healed my body and delivered me from epilepsy.

PRAYER IS THE KEY, BUT FAITH UNLOCKS DOORS

Thankfully, in 1996, I experienced a dramatic turn of events. Just after I had entered high school in September 1996, I began to experience a wave of severe epilepsy. I usually experienced seizures only once every month or go months at a time with no episodes. However, that fall, the frequency of occurence of the seizures increased to weekly, and then for the first time, twice in one day. I thought I was going to die. This all climaxed on an evening in Free Port, Grand Bahamas during my Christmas vacation when I had my last episode of epilepsy.

We were staying at the home of my cousin, Evangelist Punchetta Taylor (deceased) when I had a seizure followed by the always reliable prayer and calling on the name of Jesus by my mother. Nevertheless, Punchetta saw that I was depressed after the episode and asked me what was wrong and why I looked so sad. I told her that I was tired of the seizures and how they made me feel. I expressed to her that I have believed every prayer that went up on my behalf but God had forgotten me. I shared with her the frustration of becoming a teen and dealing with seizures and I wanted it to end, or my life to end. I continued pouring out my heart to her and sharing my disappointments and my fears about not being able to lead a normal adult life if the seizures continued.

Punchetta began to cry and said to me, "Jas, do you have enough faith to believe one more time that God can deliver you from these seizures?" I told her that I did not have enough faith but if she believed with me, maybe it would be enough. Subsequently, we prayed and I got up from the floor for the first time in a long while feeling restored.

When we returned to the TCI in 1997, I told my mother that I believed in my heart that I was healed and delivered from epilepsy, and as a result, I would no longer be taking the medication I took for eight years. The battle of wills began. My mother wanted to believe with me but was insisting that I continue to take the medication. I told mama that believing God while taking the medication was not exercising complete faith in God. Hence, despite her many pleas to me, I refused to swallow another pill.

There were many nights when she asked me if I took my pills, I lied and said 'yes' to avoid a confrontation. I remember lying down after I lied to my mother and pleading God to forgive my lie but to know that I am doing this to trust Him more than I trust the medication and my mother's intuition. The year 1997 was the first complete year that I had not experienced epileptic seizures since the age of four. Thanks be to God; 1996 was the last time I had a seizure.

The Greatest Miracle

Despite the magnitude of these experiences which developed my faith and relationship with God, they are nothing compared to the greatest healing which took place in my life; self-acceptance. I am thankful that I was relatively still young when I accepted myself for who I was and how God designed me. To be fair, people born physically perfect themselves struggle with self-acceptance; hence, you need not be too hard on yourself if you are struggling with this. There are several reasons why I consider my acceptance of myself as my greatest miracle contributing to the development of my faith.

Firstly, accepting who I was eliminated my mental state of self-pity. After spending years questioning God about why He created me the way He did and not appreciating the image I saw reflecting in the mirror, I became accustomed to pity parties and having regrets about being born. These feelings also contributed to the impact people's opinion of my appearance had on me. However, when I finally accepted that this was how God made me, many of my other problems disappeared. Secondly, this new found love for myself began to translate into other areas of my life. I started to desire to do things for myself.

I wanted to sit among large crowds and mingle with those I considered more fortunate than me (my thinking at that time). I played harder and developed an attitude of "**anything you can do, I can do better**". Moreover, my comfort level when surrounded by stronger looking people grew immensely.

Finally, once I accepted myself, I began to dream and see my abilities within my apparent disabilities. My life developed a purpose and I became determined to fulfil it. All because God brought me to a place where He healed my broken heart and self-insufficiency about my creation. He taught me how to embrace my difference and individuality and to recognize that my giftedness would only begin to make room for me and bring me before great men when I accepted that I was not only a gift but also was given talents and abilities that would positively influence the lives of other people.

There are so many examples throughout my life where God built my faith in Him due to His kindness and opened doors. This secret to getting ahead is important if you believe like I do that God makes no mistakes, especially in our creation as human beings. As obvious as it might be to many, I must still reaffirm that faith in God can move mountains in your life, but you must first believe that He can move them and He will empower you to move them as well.

Finally, only through a relationship with God, can you truly unlock your gift and divine purpose on this earth. Have faith in God, then you will be able to **find your 'abilities' within your 'disability'** and begin to transform your life and the lives of those around you.

APPLICATION

Purchase a bible or request one from your parents. This should be your personal bible since you will use it daily.

Recite these 4 Confidence Statements in the mirror daily.

1. I am healed in the name of Jesus, according to Isaiah 53:5.

2. I am made in the image of God, according to Genesis 1:27.

3. I am perfect, according to Matthew 5:48.

4. I will prosper and be in good health even as my soul prospers, according to 3 John 2.

STEP 10:

DISCOVERING THE BEST KEPT SECRETS OF GETTING AHEAD

Secret # 1: Discovering your 'Ability' within your 'Disability'

The only thing more important than your parents identifying the things you are capable of doing as early as possible is you discovering the 'abilities' within your 'disability'. No, not just in terms of daily tasks and responsibilities but rather the special talent that God deposited in you when He designed you. Each child is gifted with something they can use either as a trade or talent to transform their life and even the lives of those around them.

For example, amidst the disappointment that I once considered my physical appearance and the frustration from my symptoms of Cerebral Palsy, my mother helped me to explore the strength of my mental capacity to collect, retain and then transfer information. Both she and I were cognizant that my academic challenge was centred around my struggle to write rather than knowing what to write. Hence, from an early age, she began drilling me with speed reading and comprehension while showing me patience with the development of my writing skills. Amazingly, my greatest ability discovered then and even to this date is my written and now typewritten expression. During my later years in elementary school, I began to bury myself in books and articles about history, politics, and current affairs. This literature built my knowledge bank, as well as my oratory and public speaking skills that I would later discover, were my second greatest abilities.

Despite the consistent development of my writing skills, I still was uncomfortable standing up in front of a crowd to give a speech. Instead, I wanted to be the guy who wrote the speech for the friend and coached them on how to deliver it the way I would. However, as my self-acceptance grew, so did my confidence and my ability to deliver soliloquy after soliloquy in front of people. This is what I called **using your ability despite your disability**.

Trust His plan for your life

My first experience in using my oratory skills publicly came in March of 2001 (my final year in secondary school). I was asked by one of my favourite teachers, Mrs. Cynthia Forbes, to attend preparations for the annual Inter-High Junior Parliamentary Debate (students from various high schools would assume roles of Elected Members of Parliament) where I would simply provide support and suggestions to the participants from my school, and play a non-significant role of 'Chief Justice'. I was elated because playing the role of Chief Justice only required me to dress up in a nice suit, be escorted by two parody law enforcement officers, and be seated in a 'high seat' during the mock parliament session.

However, as you have come to expect, most stories in my life that are shared in this book take a dramatic turn just after I would have become comfortable with my present state of affairs. On the Sunday evening before the big day of the National Inter-High Junior Parliamentary Debate, one of the main participants did not show up for the final practice. The student who would play the role of Minister of Education found it convenient to miss the final and most important practice, forcing the student who was supposed to be the Speaker of the House to vacate the role and become Minister of Education.

While the reassignment of the Minister of Education was solved, it also created the need for a new Speaker of The House. Mrs. Forbes and the organizer of the event Mrs. Ruth Blackman turned to me and asked me to "just sit in the Speaker's chair during the practice runs so that the other participants would not be thrown off their game." In my heart, I felt that I was being set up but I trusted these two individuals to know that there was no way under the sun that I would be able to prepare and assume the role of Speaker of The House in less than sixteen hours.

Once more I was wrong. At the end of the practice session, I saw Mrs. Forbes and Mrs. Blackman colluding and then they both approached me smiling. Subsequently, they informed me that they wanted me to stay in the role of Speaker for the debate and that they were confident that I could do it. I was most certainly the person in that room with the least amount of confidence. I begged and pleaded with them that I had never spoken to a crowd that vast or important and that I would let them down. Nevertheless, they insisted that I could do it. The day of the debate came and I made it through. I received a number of congratulations from attendees and even the actual elected Parliamentarians were expressing how impressed they were with my performance.

From the Mountain Top

This experience boosted my confidence in public speaking and prepared me to deliver a few months later one of the greatest speeches of life; my Valedictorian's Address. One can imagine the gratitude I have to my creator for preserving the portions of my brain responsible for thinking and retention of knowledge amidst the damage done by Cerebral Palsy. I had reached the mountaintop of academic achievement in my formative education when I graduated as the Valedictorian of my high school's graduating class. However, the only thing that would be more memorable than my achievement was the unforgettable address I delivered that became known as "The Speech."

That night, I recognized the opportunity that was presented before me and spoke from my heart on a number of topics that were prevalent in my country during that period. I challenged the government and civic leaders of that period to rise to the occasion and answer the questions of my generation. Since the address was broadcasted live on national radio, I seized the moment to forever scratch my mark in my country as a conscious young man who desired more than what was currently being offered to his generation.

A SPEAKER IS BORN

One of the interesting things that spilled over from my Valedictorian's address was the newfound belief of my country that I was a great speaker. Subsequently, I was invited to participate in a competition to represent the Turks & Caicos Islands in St. Kitts at the Caribbean Parliamentary Association Conference. I did not win the competition, but Mrs. Ruth Blackman insisted that I attend the conference as an observer. This was a great opportunity for me as I would have my first trip to the Eastern Caribbean as well as experience the pride and joy of being an ambassador for the Turks & Caicos Islands.

The experience from that trip provided me with enough memories to last a lifetime but it was eclipsed when I was informed a year later that I would once more represent my country at the same conference in Tortola, British Virgin Islands as the senior youth parliamentarian. When we arrived in Tortola, we were the first youth parliamentarians to reach from among the seventeen participating countries in the West Indies. After enjoying the hospitality of some of the friendliest people I had ever met, the Youth Parliamentary Debate (which was the highlight of the entire conference) was drawing near and the participants were separated into two groups; government members and opposition members. Before I left my country, I was informed that I would be a member of the government for the mock parliamentary debate, so I went prepared to make a valuable contribution to the team.

Those experiences representing my country changed my life significantly because it put me on a path towards using my abilities and talents to live my dreams. From that point forward, my gifts began to make room for me and I started thinking more about what I was capable of doing rather than those things I could not do. I refuse to believe that this concept only applies to me. No matter how you may feel about your disposition in life, there is something within you that can be used to impact your life positively. The task is yours to **identify, accept it, and then seek to develop it**. From personal testimony, the more I used my abilities to affect positive change, the less I was viewed or lived as a person with a disability. Believe me, when you reach a place in life where you can fully enjoy your life and you are no longer severely impacted by your physical or cognitive disabilities, you will have reached the plateau of "dreaming beyond your diagnosis".

Secret #2: To Grow; You Must Learn to Forgive

From the minute some people realize you are different, they will make it their business to hurt you or make life difficult for you. Then there are those who ignorantly say hurtful or inappropriate things to you because they could not see the potential in you that needed nurturing and support. Nevertheless, you must learn to defy these people's desire for your life without hating them or holding resentment against them in your heart for the things they have said or done to you. Trust me, I know this can be so difficult but it is critical for your personal growth and development that you forgive them.

Let me share a story with you. This story is one of the most difficult ones for me to write for several reasons. Firstly, some memories are very painful to revisit and when you share intimate experiences of your life which involves your family, you can get backlash as your reward. Secondly, I am not writing this from a place of unforgiveness or malice rather than a place of healing and appreciation. Moreover, my intention is to encourage a family to not make the mistakes mine made and to encourage someone who has experienced or will experience what I did not to become bitter but better.

One of the greatest challenges of my childhood was being fully accepted by my father's family. I knew they loved me but many of the experiences I had growing up indicated to me that they wished I was what people would call 'normal'. There were several times when my grandmother and grandfather would accuse me of seeking pity because I asked for help with getting dressed (for the record it took me 15 years before I was able to button my shirt by myself) or doing something I did not have the confidence to do with both my hands. As a child, I listened to some of my father's siblings and my grandmother share their opinions of the way my mother took extra care and protected me in a way that inferred that my mom was raising me to be dependent on other people.

There were many times I left my grandmother's house crying and telling my mama of my experiences (I will not get into details) and expressed to her that I did not want to go back but mama only comforted me and said "Jas, don't worry. Everything will be fine". My mama would always encourage me not to be resentful but keep believing in myself. I remember one day while walking home from grandmother's house, I prayed and asked God to give me favour and a life that would make my family see me as a gift from God, and He answered that prayer. While going through those moments, it was painful and there were times I did not enjoy being around my father's family. But I grew and they also grew. Hence, I had to forgive the hurt and ignorant things that were said to me not just in order to love them, but also so I could learn to love myself.

I had to do the same thing when I returned from college and encountered some adults and former children (now adults) who had bullied or teased me when I was growing up. I learned that sometimes, to heal and grow, **you must forgive people** and especially those who might never say sorry or acknowledge that they were wrong about you. Furthermore, when you forgive the hurts and offences of people, it allows you to leave those hurts in the past. Until you do, you will never be able to fully embrace your future and what it has in store for you.

My life has taught me many lessons but one of the most important lessons is this: people can only try to hold you back in life by the negative words they speak over your life or the obstacles they put in your way. However, you keep yourself back when you accept those negative words or stop seeking ways around or through those obstacles set by others. **Get up, forgive, and keep moving.**

SECRET #3: YOU HAVE TO PUT IN OVERTIME ALL THE TIME

When you realize that your disability creates challenges for you, besides facing those challenges and discovering your abilities within your disability, one of the most important secret ingredients to getting ahead is that you will have to put in overtime, all the time. Truth be told, this secret applies to people with no disability or special needs. However, it is even more paramount for someone with a special need to be prepared to work doubly hard to achieve their goals in life. Your attitude must take on the persona of an unrelenting engine that just keeps accelerating even when other cars seem to be cruising or parked.

For example, from the moment my Nana (Yvette Gardiner) sat me down and explained to me that I could not afford to play around with academic work, explaining to me that my physical limitations would narrow the field of employment for me if I was thinking about doing manual labour, I knew I would have to put in some overtime in life. Nana made me understand I had to use my brain and let it earn me an "office job in an air-conditioned comfortable environment" (her exact words). She stressed to me the need to focus on my studies and not to slack my riding because I was not strong enough to get by on laborious jobs one after the other. In my reflection, I can honestly state that this heart to heart with Nana opened my eyes and gave me a reality check. Since that conversation at age eleven, I have developed an "overtime all the time" approach to living because my experiences have taught me that in life, few might have sympathy for you, but none will give you a free pass or a head start. Hence, **you must put in the extra work.**

The extra work is what I did to maintain the top average in my class amidst stiff competition on the way to being the Valedictorian. A friend and classmate, Dr. Jameko Harvey, pushed me to the extreme because we both wanted to be number one. He was gifted in the sciences and technical vocational areas and I focused on the arts and linguistics. Our back and forth battle culminated with the final exit mock exam. Despite being devastated emotionally by the loss of my father in January 2001, I had to find a way to regain my focus and finish strong. There were many nights in which sleep was calling me but I fought it because I did not want Jameko to beat me and even heard voices in my head telling me "Jas, you better get up. Jameko is studying. Jas, you have to work harder than Jameko".

Not to mention, I always remembered a verse from a poem taken from "The Ladder of St. Augustine" by Henry Wadsworth Longfellow, drilled in me by my father:

The heights by great men reached and kept

Were not attained by sudden flight,

But they, while their companions slept,

Were toiling upward in the night.

And with every recollection of that verse, I got another boost of inner motivation and continued to put in the overtime. In the end (as you would have previously read), I beat Jameko and was the Valedictorian. However, I did not stop there. I took that driven attitude with me to college and throughout my career. To this day, I continue to put extra (and sometimes undue) pressure on myself to excel. Because I still live as if I am being chased for the prize or if I am still in the fight of my life to achieve the goals I have set for myself. That is not to say that there will not be disappointments or setbacks in life, but never let them occur because you did not put in the overtime.

Places you may go because you said 'yes'

For instance, I put everything I could into a campaign for College Student Union President. My campaign did activities never before done during a student union election; held campaign rallies on campus, printed t-shirts, created campaign music and a detailed manifesto and excited the campus base for the first time in decades. My opponent was failing academically and did not even print a poster visible on campus. However, on the day of the election, he snuck into the polling area (which was the campus cafeteria) and solicited votes from students who were not a part of the election activities. Although during the candidate's meeting we were told that we had to stay two hundred feet from the polling area, he was allowed there because he was the establishment's choice. At the end of the counting of the ballots, my opponent beat me by nearly two hundred votes.

I was devastated and very disappointed because I knew I ran the better campaign and did it on a platform of class and conviction for change, but still lost. The irony of this story is that in less than twenty-four hours, I had to get ready to compete against the same individual in a speech competition on campus. Well, guess what? I won the competition and the three hundred dollars cash prize as well as a pizza party for my education club colleagues. He placed almost last, and while it was not as satisfying as winning the Presidency, it was a consolation gift for me.

If you thought that was rough, try running for public office during your country's general elections. The more the campaign progressed, the more I began to desire victory for my supporters more than for myself. I found out that inspiration is like a contagious disease that spreads from one person to the next. Did I put everything I had into that campaign? Yes, I did. I wanted to make sure that every voter in my country understood why I offered myself for elected office. I wanted them to make an informed decision and judge me on my character and shared convictions rather than the political colours or platitudes we have clung to over these many years.

I was unsuccessful in my bid for elected office in the 2016 general elections and it was a disappointment that I had to accept as 'divine intervention'. I was disappointed because my decision to run was never about what I wanted for myself but rather, what I wanted for my country. It was not my time to become a member of parliament. But it was my time to introduce myself to this country and give them a glimpse of what was possible in politics. It was my time to inspire my generation and those to follow that "**even though defeat/ failure may seem imminent, you must still run your race because winning is not everything.**" You will not be able to grow from experiences in life without some disappointments and setbacks. Pick yourself up and keep running and keep putting in the overtime because one day it will pay off.

Interestingly enough, three years later in the Turks & Caicos Civil Service (Public Service), I was nominated to run for President of the Civil Service Association. At first, I told them that after my college and general elections experience, I was done with running for public office for now. However, after the overwhelming nomination votes from all over the country came in, I decided to make another run and as usual, put in the overtime with my campaign. Thankfully, and after two unsuccessful bids, I won a race in elected office. On June 24th, 2019, I was elected as the President of the country's Civil Service Association by capturing nearly sixty-five percent (65%) of the votes cast for President among three other candidates. Although being criticized by other candidates for going 'overboard' with a campaign website, an original campaign song, printed flyers, and radio interviews, I made no apologies because I was simply putting in 'overtime' and this time the overtime resulted in victory.

Moreover, the fact that you can read these words is evidence of me putting in overtime. 'Overtime' allowed me to write, then learn to type, and eventually inspired me to put this book together. Basically, I am living proof that putting in overtime all the time pays off.

Secret #4: Amidst Success: Stay Humble

One of the most sacred quotes I can recall my great grandmother Roselyn Gardiner (deceased) saying to us as children was "a humble child tastes the grace of God". It was ingrained into me from that time and thankfully it has never left me as an adult. There are so many people who have risen above their challenges and attained greatness in life. However, there are so many of those people who have developed a lofty and arrogant spirit as if they were always great or were born having already accomplished everything. This attitude often leads to pride, and you must always remember that 'pride always comes before the fall'; hence, amidst your past, present, and future success, you must **remain humble**. There are three lessons in humility I have learnt over the years and I will share them with you.

Lesson #1: The first lesson in humility I learnt was knowing how to ask for and accept help. Because I was accustomed to so many people looking at me as a disabled person and as someone who was weak, it built a stupid sense of pride in me at times when I undertook tasks too great for me and did not want to ask for help. Additionally, I recall going to a store and the shopkeeper putting a small message in my bag to assist me, and instead of appreciating the help, I viewed it as pity and insisted that I could do it myself. After repeated protests, the storekeeper stopped trying to assist me with packaging my small items. Guess what happened later? There came a point where I wanted the assistance and it was not offered.

As I grew and went away to school and developed into an independent living young man, I continued to struggle with accepting help from people. I remember foolishly feeling as if I was being patronized when people would leave a door open for me or gave up a seat on the bus so I could sit. Thankfully, as I matured I began to swallow my foolish pride and accepted help from people whether I needed it or not. Why? Because I realized people are not obligated to help you; it is a choice they make.

Secondly, when we pray to God for help or favour in our lives, He sends it in the form of the people being His hands extended. Finally, I began to see that one of the few perks of being physically different at times is that it positions you to receive preferential treatment. My advice to you, **when it is offered, take it!**

Lesson #2: My second lesson in humility is to never use the pain experienced because of what others did to you as an excuse to inflict pain on other people. Pain is an unfortunate but necessary element in life. However, how you respond to it is what will determine your destiny. It was and sometimes still tempting for me to be bitter and seek petty revenge on people or relatives who I knew tormented me or spoke negative, disparaging words into my life to make me feel defeated, especially considering how successful I have become thus far. Moreover, if I behaved towards them the same way they behaved towards me, how does that make me different? Instead, I have learnt to appreciate my growth as well as theirs in recognizing that I am an overcomer and stubborn go-getter. When the opportunity comes to help those who hurt you, take it, and **help those individuals**. Believe me, accepting your help might be much more awkward and difficult for them than offering it might be for you.

Lesson #3: Finally, never, never, ever forget your creator and where He has brought you from. There will be moments in your life when you have made so much progress in pursuing your dreams that you will see the way people look at you change over time. This is a great feeling but also very dangerous. When people genuinely celebrate your milestones and call you a champion after every major victory, it is easy for you to develop pride and self-glorification and take the credit for the miracles that have transformed your life. Let me share something with you which speaks to this sentiment I am trying to express. During my third year in college, I was coming off a successful representation of my country at a regional Caribbean Parliamentary Conference, popularity soaring high despite my failed bid for Student Union Presidency, and had become a household name in most college social circles.

I was no longer the shy and insecure little boy ready to cry at every insult about my physical difference. One morning I woke up feeling as if I was on the top of the world. I did not pray or acknowledge God for giving me a new day and went on the bus as I usually did to get to my classes. When I got on the bus that morning, I was full of confidence, but suddenly a feeling of fear and insecurity came over me. I began to shake and sweat like I was having a seizure. Passengers kept looking at me and asking if I was doing ok. Despite my efforts to convince them that I was feeling fine, they began to press the driver to take me to the hospital. Thankfully, he was familiar with me and recalled my initial days of catching the bus, and how I used to be so nervous. Hence, he told the concerned passengers to stand down.

When I arrived at the college campus, I immediately went into the bathroom to compose myself. I began to cry and did not understand why I felt so unbalanced that morning. Then, like a lightbulb came on in my head, I realized I have not acknowledged God for a while and I heard these words spoken to me, "Jas, who do you think you are? It was me who created you and favoured you. Don't you ever forget me". I fell to the ground in humility and prayed with tears in my eyes, asking

God to forgive my pride. That was the last morning I woke up with that attitude. No matter where God takes you or what He has allowed you to achieve, never make your success all about you. His design in your life is for a specific purpose and ultimately to give Him glory. **Stay humble** and you will be exalted and promoted from peak to peak.

Secret #5: Never Stop Dreaming

As I write this final chapter and excerpt on dreams, I am overwhelmed with emotions for a number of reasons. Firstly, I can recall a period in my life when I did not have any dreams or thoughts of life as an adult. That period was marred with self-pity and disgust over the circumstances of my birth, accusing God of being unfair to me, and frustration with self-acceptance. I wanted nothing in life except to be like others – yes, that was my only dream and the only desire for my life at that time. Some thirty-five years later, I have so many dreams for my life that I had to start writing them down. Your dreams do not start when you sleep, instead, your dreams start when you live, and not just live but live with meaning and purpose with a determination to defy people's expectations and limitations for your life.

As I have illustrated in the previous pages of this book, my life was one of struggle, confrontation, hard work, and then victory. That being said, I define 'a dream' as any goal you have set for your life and your plans to attain them. Just like Joseph in the Bible, people will often oppose you because they see that you are special and become frustrated with you when your dreams supersede the dreams they have for their own lives. Hence, they begin to plot your demise and conspire to destroy you, believing it will destroy your dreams. However, newsflash! If your dreams are planted by God, nothing men can do will stop them from coming true. Instead, their actions against you often inadvertently further repositions you on a path of achieving those dreams. If you are having doubts in your heart, study the life of Biblical Joseph who went from being a slave to a prime minister.

I think it has been established that I have learnt many valuable lessons in this miraculous, highly favoured life I have lived. However, very few lessons were as powerful as this one: your greatest offense to people is when through trusting in God, you have lived your dreams in defiance of what they think you should be and how you should live. Not to mention if you have been designed physically different, they tend to add more barriers and control to your life. So, if you have not learnt anything from me, please learn this: **under no circumstances can you let other people control your dreams or the possibilities of your life**. I pray for your sake, that you have been fortunate to have a supportive and caring mother as I did, one whose love and dedication to your dreams will one day inspire you to write about them the same way I have done.

If that has not been your experience, don't bury your head in the sand. Instead, pick yourself up and carry on. God will put people in your life to provide you with the similar support my mother, Maurine, my Nana, and many others provided me.

Finally, there might be people who after reading this book, may conclude that I did not really live life as a person with a disability or special need, and the truth of the matter, your perspective might be correct. However, it was not because I did not have physical handicaps due to the circumstances of my birth, neither was it because I had a wealth of resources to facilitate my inclusion in school or community. Instead, the circumstances of the era I was born and raised in, as well as the miracle of my birth, never afforded my mother and me a proper diagnosis or correct terminology for my medical condition. Therefore, in the absence of a medical label, we fought to live life like everyone else, without labels. Perhaps had I known my medical diagnosis from birth, I might have used it as an excuse to underachieve and not dream.

Thankfully, times have changed and there has been more education on the subject as well as exposure for special needs individuals which have provided better assessment and diagnosis for children. Hence, more than likely, you would have been diagnosed and have been explained the characteristics of your disability. Nevertheless, don't use it as an excuse to underachieve and fail to dream. Instead, follow my pattern and **live your life without labels** because a diagnosis does not have to be a death sentence. A medical diagnosis is a medical explanation for a condition you have and guides the physician in treating you, not how you treat yourself. Moreover, your dream is how you choose to live with that condition. Simply put, '**dream beyond your diagnosis**'.

APPLICATION

1) Write the names of 3 people you need to forgive.

a. _____

b. _____

c. _____

2) Write 3 goals that you would like to accomplish in the next 5 years.

a. _____

b. _____

c. _____

2) Write 3 ways you will change the world!

a. _____

b. _____

c. _____

Final Remarks

To the Villiage:

To my Uniquely-abled Friend:

REFLECTION

REFLECTION

REFLECTION

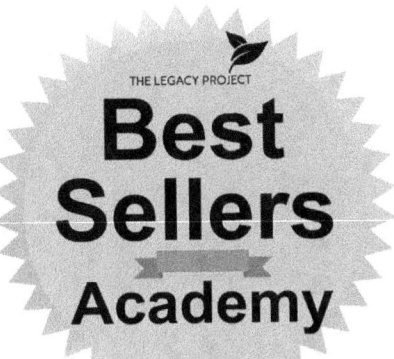

This book was published with the support of The Bestsellers Academy.

Do you have a book inside of you?

Let us get your story out of your belly and into an international bestselling book!

Phone: 1-868-374-7441

Email: success@thebestsellersacademy.com

Website: TheBestsellersAcademy.com

www.ingramcontent.com/pod-product-compliance
Lightning Source LLC
Chambersburg PA
CBHW070252220526
45465CB00004B/1586